RAGE RISING - MY WALK THROUGH THE DARK TUNNEL OF ANGER

BONNIE LACY

FROSTING ON THE CAKE PRODUCTIONS

*I don't write to change the world.
I write to change me.*

CONTENTS

Introduction	vii
Ted Dekker's Book Excerpt	xi
Vision	xiii

PART I
THE SET-UP

1. Rich's Accident	3
2. September 2002 - Jennifer Gets Sick	13
3. Me	23
4. Jeff at Teen Challenge	33
5. Mom	39
6. Harriet	49

PART II
RECOVERY

7. Bridge to Recovery	57
8. Jeff in My Face	65
9. Christ-Life	69
10. Take Care of ME	73
11. Counseling	77
12. Strong Tower	81
13. Joy - Or Lack of It	85
14. Writing	95
Epilogue	105
Acknowledgements	107
Stay Connected	109

INTRODUCTION

I can feel it brewing.

It feels like a fist in my gut—fingers twisting and writhing—until it has to explode. This isn't the old butterflies in my stomach feeling. And somehow those fingers connect to my eyes, because I want to weep. A monster resides in my heart and is pounding its way through to my thinking, my decisions and my mouth. And what comes out of my mouth are words ready to stab anyone within range.

Just being honest.

Rage Rising may seem like a strong title for a book, but rage or anger is a powerful emotion. And it's not that I want to puke this stuff out here. I want everybody to think I'm this nice lady who writes and doodles. Plays with grandkids. Bakes brownies for people out of the goodness ... of ... of my heart? (See above about what's in my heart! Hint: a monster! If you're a visual person, and most people are, getting a visual of a monster baking brownies is almost comical—depending on the day.)

My words, my attitudes, have probably done more damage than I could ever imagine.

But I'm getting ahead of the ... story.

I'm reading Brené Brown's book, *Daring Greatly* and on page 60, she says, "Only when we're brave enough to explore the darkness will we discover the infinite power of our light."

Brave? Uh. No.

Explore the darkness ... I guess that's why I'm writing this book. Hopefully, I will find who I am meant to be. Also hopefully, who I'm supposed to be is not the angry woman I have become.

Brené wrote on page 61, "We can't let ourselves be seen if we're terrified by what people might think."

I am.

Terrified of what people might think. If they only knew what my thoughts have been and are—what my insides must look like.

But I am even more terrified to stay in this mess.

Farther down on page 61, "But if we don't come to terms with our shame, our struggles, we start believing that there's something wrong with us—that we're bad, flawed, not good enough—and even worse, we start acting on those beliefs."

Acting on those beliefs. I have acted on the darkness—spewing out words of anger. If you follow the steps through anger, they start with offense, resentment, bitterness ... on through anger, violence, murder.

Murder?

I'm hoping to find, in writing this book, my way out of that tunnel of anger, and that I will continue to heal.

By the way, I don't write to change the world.

I write to change me.

Sorry.

If that sounds selfish. It's not. It's all about survival.

But I also hope that maybe someone who reads this will be changed, too. Is that you?

I hope you will read and interact with me. Email me. What are your thoughts? Together we might open those memories and wounds, and expose them to the Light.

And heal.

I'll go first.

Anger is what fed me back then. I'm sure it had been lurking underneath before, but a chain of events within two and a half years jump-started the deadly percolating of anger and fear deep within me: my daughter was very sick with West Nile, my husband had an accident where the other guy was committing suicide and was okay with taking my Dearly Beloved with him, Mom was dying of lung cancer, and a son was addicted to cocaine—all within just over two years.

That's when I stepped into that dark tunnel.

If I'd known then what I know now, would I have changed anything? What did I learn?

But I'm getting ahead of myself.

From Journal 1/24/2018: Journal entries. Raw emotion—not brilliant writing. They were never meant to be shared. But here they are: raw and unedited. I open them up to you, allowing you to feel what I felt.

So, how do I do this?

How do I puke this anger out?

I have my *second* pile of Kleenex beside me on the table—I had a cold.

Right.

How do I produce this book?

I want to give people hope but I want it to be different. Not the everyday self-help book. I want to make a difference in someone's life—give them hope—change their trajectory. I don't have three steps to recovery or a step-by-step guide to overcoming anger.

That's not what this is.

This is one woman's story of her walk through that slimy sludge lining a dark tunnel of anger.

And to be honest, I go back into that awful tunnel—not because I want to—but because it's home. I have to learn to take a different path.

I used to be scared of what might lurk under my bed when I was a kid—I remember! I'd lie in bed at night, scared of what might pop up, terrified of the unknown, the imagined. The unseen.

Until I'd finally fall asleep.

Rarely did I venture downstairs to wake my parents. Probably because I knew it was foolish, childish.

But was it?

Maybe that's why I'm so drawn to tunnels, underground caves, sink holes. Because they feel comfortable—places where I can hide, where I don't have to deal with people, or life. Hide away in the dark, in a place that should scare me. Maybe what was *in* me was scarier than what might, or might not have been under my bed.

If this story gets too close to you—too intense or scary—don't feel bad about throwing the book away. I intend to be honest.

That's scary.

TED DEKKER'S BOOK EXCERPT

Speaking of scary, I think I have read every one of Ted Dekker's books, unless they aren't out yet!

He speaks (or writes) in my language.

<u>Showdown</u>. Page 23—"The flame's light lapped at the wall's moss-covered stones. Moisture seeped through the rock and dripped unevenly on the cobblestones, sending echoes down the black hall."

Page 24—"Water dripped incessantly, and the worms slid along moist walls made slimy by their mucus. Beyond thirty feet, the tunnel faded into blackness."

Icky tunnels—I get that. My insides felt just like that—icky, nasty.

I get the stones, the rock—I literally shut everyone out who wanted to help, especially my sister, my kids. But because of anger, I built my tunnel, enclosed it brick by brick until no one could get inside.

I closed myself off.

My pain was shut inside where it would fester, where pus could build and get nasty.

Slimy.

My insides ached from holding it all in.

I still trusted God, I just couldn't *give* it to him. I didn't open it all up because I was afraid I'd never stop crying—or that I'd die. I had to hold it together.

What would people think if I fell apart?

I was the one everyone came to for help.

But, I wasn't the one who had West Nile or lung cancer. I didn't have to deal with the pain of addictions or withdrawals. I didn't have re-occurring nightmares of car headlights aiming straight for my truck.

Then why did all this affect *me* so deeply?

Maybe it was because I couldn't *fix* them. I couldn't make the West Nile go away.

I couldn't make my Mom well—she was dying.

I had to lay down my hopes and dreams for my son's life.

And I couldn't protect my husband from a man who had been running from the law, committing atrocities and who was willing to take my husband down with him.

The man died.

My husband, by the Grace of God, lived.

VISION

Back in December 2000, I had a vision. In it I was dressed in a long lavender skirt and vest over a T-shirt—the same as I had on in the physical realm—and I was standing up on a high plain or plateau. I was looking far off in many different directions, as an eagle would, the wind lifting my hair off my face, fluttering my skirt against my legs. It was as if I was a TV camera on a wheeled dolly, panning, picturing a panoramic view.

An eagle can see for miles—searching for prey, food, enemies, or upcoming storms and, like an eagle, one of the wonderful things the Holy Spirit does is to help us see things to come—things in the distance. I believe we also have the ability to discern upcoming events as Elijah could sense (1 Kings 18:41), either the coming of a storm or a blessing, "for there is the sound of abundance of rain."

Rain is a blessing, but dark storm clouds precede it.

I love storm clouds, lightning and thunder.

I can still see that vision. Feel the wind flapping my skirt. Still see things, events in the distance.

As the vision progressed, the Lord spoke words to me, but I can't remember them right now.

It's okay.

Those words are still with me. He is the Word and the Word is alive. He is in me and I am in Him. So I have the words He spoke, still active and living inside of me today, whether I remember them or not.

Again, if I could have seen every situation back then, the dark clouds forming, would I have changed anything? *Could I have?*

Maybe.

My decision should have been to react with grace and peace.

But I reacted with hate and rage.

I am reminded that an eagle often flies into the storm and flows with the wind currents.

I didn't.

I built a wall and hid behind it.

If I would have engaged with the vision, gone to those heights far away, would I have seen what was to happen?

I didn't know what I know now.

PART I
THE SET-UP

1
RICH'S ACCIDENT

That Early Morning Call

It was a cold December morning in 2003, the day after Christmas, when my phone rang.

"Bon?" My husband, Rich, choked on the words. "Bon. I'm okay."

Any conversation that starts off with "I'm okay" can't be good.

"Yeah?" I was still groggy and my head dropped back onto the pillow. I squinted at the clock. 6 something a.m.—hard to see. Good grief, he had just left on a haul to take classic cars to a customer. I must have fallen back into a deep sleep.

"I was in an accident. But I'm okay." He still sounded strange, like there was a catch in his voice, but it was early and maybe he had caught a cold.

I still hadn't figured out that *he had just been in an accident!*

Honestly? I was thinking I could go back to sleep for a little bit. I was still exhausted after all the celebrations. The kids were still home. Our first grandchild was here, probably close to waking, his baby tummy growling.

But something or Someone gave me the boot I needed to get out of bed. I finally got the idea that this was real and I needed to get up and dress and go.

Rich told me where he was and I hung up. I probably put on the clothes I had worn the day before—my Christmas Day attire. From there on, things are kind of a blur, but I definitely remember fumbling with my car keys. If I had to wake kids to have them move their vehicles so I could get out, I can't remember.

Barely daylight, I started off to where I thought Rich was, but met an emergency unit. At about that same time, I got a call on my cell phone (thank God we had those then). It was a friend who was an EMT and I believe a fireman.

"Where are you?"

"I'm just past the big corner."

"Turn around and go back to town. If you met the emergency unit, Rich is in it and they are taking him to the hospital."

Hospital. I think that's when I finally woke up.

His voice got louder. "Don't come out here to the scene." He cleared his throat. "Don't come out here."

Hospital

Rich's memory of the hospital: vitals, drug and alcohol testing, cleaning up where he had been pelted with glass, flushing his eyes out.

He said it was confirmed at the hospital that the man who had caused the accident was dead.

My memory of the hospital? Nothing. I can't remember anything about the room, the people, the smells.

Nothing.

I recently asked my son-in-law what he remembers. He does remember the hospital. "Rich was joking with the nurses," he said.

After an accident? Normal for Rich Lacy.

But I only remember the hallway in the ER. Not the room where Rich was.

You would think the shock of hearing about the accident, seeing my Dearly Beloved with glass cuts peppering his face and neck, would be an in-your-face recollection, but it isn't there. I don't have that picture. I don't have that memory. Or is it buried deep under daily life—work, writing, hugging grandkids? Seriously. I cannot bring it out no matter what.

Maybe I'm not supposed to.

I'M A HARD-CORE JOURNALING ADDICT. I just counted all my journals—*filled* journals—not pretty ones gifted to me. Not clean, blank journals waiting in the cupboard to be opened and destroyed by me. I'm talking about completely messed-up spiral notebooks, ragged edged moleskins, dirty doodled-on-and-in sketchbooks. They total forty-seven. I just started forty-eight!

I have spent a small fortune on them, some expensive beauties—I have a leather 8 x 10 cover and I can switch out the insides when I fill them. Interesting though: I usually grab a black 8 x 10 spiral sketchbook from Walmart. The old spiral notebooks are leftover from my kids' school days. I kept them, tore out pages they had used for history notes and doodling. I have scribbled on the rest.

Miserly. I could be a direct descendant of Ebenezer Scrooge. (Look for my book, Cash Envelopes: You've Never Had So Much Money, due out in 2018.)

I have dug through each journal. (I know—who has that kind of time? But I had to read each one. I had to see, to know. Maybe as a form of healing? Hope in remembering?) I flipped to the dates around December 26, 2003.

There is a huge gap in my writing from December 21, 2003 until February 29, 2004.

You'd think that I would have written pages and pages about that morning of the accident: the sounds, the smells, visuals. The aftermath.

I didn't even reminisce about Christmas. That holiday had to have been memorable with our first grandson: baby giggles, drools, cuteness.

Nothing.

There was nothing. No comments. No descriptions.

Nothing.

And I journal everything.

Scene of the Accident

The scene of the accident was only about ten miles from our house.

Rich was discharged after a couple hours and he wanted to go back.

Go back?

Either he had a secret Masters Degree in Psychology that told him to face his fears, or something called to him from the scene. Our fireman friend had explicitly told me over the phone to not go out there.

But we did. We went out there—kids, too. Not baby.

We have many photos taken by the kids, so they help in triggering memories. What follows is what I do remember, but just random thoughts and observations.

Parts and debris were scattered all over the road and ditches. Have you seen photos of tornado damage? Yeah. Wreckage all over.

Interesting, there's no traffic.

Oh.

It's all blocked off.

And it was going to be blocked for over five hours. I don't even want to think about the grumbling and cussing of the people in vehicles stopped by the deputies—how their day had been interrupted, their busy lives messed with, making them late for an appointment. Yes, I'm being snarky—knowing what my *own* response would have been and would probably be today if I had been the one waiting in line for hours to get to my hair appointment or probably having to potty!

This is where things get interesting—well, it's all overwhelming to say the least—but when I talked to Dearly Beloved recently about the accident, he swears he didn't go back to the site.

And I am bet-you-sure he and I walked around there together.

Photos tell the truth. One picture shows Dearly Beloved's bald head close to the driver side window that is now at ground level, peering inside. Right beside him, son Jeff can be seen—his yellow hat on his head.

Trauma does things to the memory. It quietly encapsulates

those dark pictures so we cannot revisit them until we are healing—like now.

Or maybe never.

Maybe it doesn't matter.

When I showed Rich the photos, he had to look closely at the one with Jeff to make sure it was really him. He truly didn't have that memory, or else it was covered up. When I showed him another picture of him walking the site with two deputies, all searching the ground, it triggered the memory. He remembered.

The kids had showed up by then. They are all adults, but it was still hard to take in. We walked all over the site.

Well, not on *that* side of the highway.

Men—friends—all firemen or EMTs were working to clean up the debris and clear the road so they could open it to traffic.

The car that had caused the accident was off limits in the other ditch.

I heard the words, "He's dead."

What?

But my mind couldn't go there right then.

People were over there, but they guided me away.

Not that I wanted to see a dead man, but it was all so strange. So disorienting. I've seen accidents along the roads before—we all have—but nothing like this.

I had never walked on site. I had never before experienced an accident up close, walking around mangled vehicle parts and tires and glass.

This accident involved my husband.

He could have died there.

Sequence of Events

The rest of the story.

According to reports, the man who caused the accident had been doing nasty things the night before. The Sheriff's Department had been searching for him all night apparently and finally found him at the scene of the accident.

Rich's memories are of headlights moving toward him from out of the dark, seemingly right in his path. Surely the lights would go back into the other lane.

Was the guy asleep?

Drunk?

But they didn't veer into the other lane, so Rich swerved to his right to miss the car. He could see it was a car now.

It was going fast when it hit Rich's 1 Ton 2001 Chevy Duramax, and the impact sheared off the driver side wheels—front wheel and back duals—making the truck slam over on its side, still moving fast, driver side now sliding against the ground. At that point, glass had shattered out from the windows, pelting Rich's face and neck.

The trailer carrying two classic cars kept pushing ahead over the truck, jackknifing, landing on top of the truck, with Rich still in it.

He astoundingly remembers Peace.

Peace.

He just held on—along for the ride.

He remembers coming out of a kind of dreamland—from a different world. He didn't black out, though. He climbed out through the drivers' side window, then realized his info and wallet were still in the truck so he had to climb back in.

I'm not sure who called the accident in. I assume a nearby farmer who had heard the impact called 911.

When the emergency unit arrived, a good friend hugged Rich. He shouldn't have survived. Even though he had been up and walking around, they got him on a back-board, stabilized and into the ambulance, taking his vitals.

The sheriff's department had been tracking the man all night.

They found their man.

Rich walked away, full of glass, but alive.

The other man didn't walk away.

Me

Numb.

That's the only way I can describe ... me.

I remember walking around, listening to Rich talk to deputies, firemen. Seeing our kids there. I remember faces, a firefighter friend who helped me maintain my car when Rich was out of town. The friend was also the one who had called me earlier and told me to follow the emergency unit. All their faces were full of concern and total disbelief at the visuals all around them and what had transpired.

I can go back there right now and place myself on the site, walking. In a fog.

But I still can't go to the hospital in my memories.

Back then we had one grandson. The day before, our son-in-law had been sitting on a rocking chair at our Christmas celebration, holding that precious baby. In the photo, our grandson is so cute, smiling, drooling. Happy. Our son-in-law is smiling.

We have another photo, from the day of the accident, with Rich at home sitting on that same rocker, holding our grandson.

But in those photos, Rich didn't look at the camera in any of the three shots. Just looked down. I can't even remember whose idea it was to take that shot or set it up.

Who wanted the photo?

Rich?

Me?

I can't remember.

But the look on Rich's face makes me want to weep. What are the thoughts traveling through his mind right then, hours after ...

He must be numb.

I have no words to describe his expression. Lifeless comes to mind. There are no tears. No expression. No emotion.

What he just went through.

The vivid images still haunt him day and night.

Even to this day he comments on the exact spot where it all took place as we drive by.

Almost every time.

2
SEPTEMBER 2002 - JENNIFER GETS SICK

How Do I Tell This?

We all have stories we could tell. Your spouse gets laid off. A child becomes very sick. Someone has to have surgery. A hurricane hits hard. An accident.

If you sat down to start the process of journaling or writing your story, where would *you* begin?

I know. Overwhelming.

Most stories span years. Mine do.

I asked God, "How do I tell this?"

His words: "Start at the beginning. Tell your story."

Ugh. That covers ten or more journals, full of daily rantings and puke-it-out-entries. Pages and pages.

And pages.

I gathered them all—tricky, since we have moved and stashed anything we didn't immediately need in a storage garage. Boxes and boxes of ... yeah. Probably stuff we don't need. (That's another chapter! Or another book!)

I figured out what years I needed and gathered the journals, along with a stack of sticky notes. If you have ever journaled and gone back to read those scribblings, you know that sometimes your "I'm gonna get this done today" voice is slowed or stopped altogether. You land on an entry that is so profound or painful that as you read it again and again, the memory washes over you.

One such entry is from January 2001 about a dream I had. Without boring you with the whole thing, at the end of the dream I was caught up in grief so deep that I was sobbing, apparently for my daughter. When I woke, I could still hear the sobs. I asked the Lord what it meant. He said, "She won't die, but she has to go through it and learn to move on." I had written the Bible verse, "I can do all things through Christ Who strengthens me." Phil. 4:13.

Easy to say then.

Before.

In January 2001.

September 2002, a year and a half later, my daughter got very sick.

Prophetic? Maybe.

A warning? Probably.

Sometimes I do go back and read a journal, but I hadn't gone back to this one.

Until now.

Journals

Rich's accident happened on our daughter Jenn's birthday and I don't remember even acknowledging it or her. We were all so caught up with the accident.

Almost a year and a half before the accident, there had been a phone call, too.

That phone call.

Jenn and her husband, and Rich and I, had been to a wedding Saturday night in September, 2002. She had been a bridesmaid and soloist, so it had been especially busy for her. When they were at our house Sunday evening, she seemed tired and her eyes looked funny. I remember asking if she felt okay. She admitted she was tired and had kind of a headache. Hopefully she'd get some rest that night before going back to work on Monday.

Monday brought the call. She said she had a major migraine and would I take her to the doctor?

"Absolutely. I'll be over to pick you up."

It was only a few miles away so it didn't take me long, but I'm sure it seemed forever to her. I didn't even take a notebook or journal. We didn't expect anything out of the ordinary. She just needed rest.

Like I said before. It had been a busy weekend.

JOURNAL: February 19, 2003

Doctor appointment for Jenn: MS or cystic fibrosis?

Nurses said she was primed to have babies because when they did the spinal tap, she was a trooper.

I found notes in this journal entry from a doctor appointment. "Could have been mono. Not West Nile."

Her symptoms were all over the place, literally.

What she was tested for over the next couple years: Meningitis, brain tumor, Crohn's disease, colitis, MS, cystic fibrosis,

Lyme disease, among many other things. They just didn't know.

I saw her cry only a few times. One was the day the Infectious Disease doctor decided to test for HIV. If she had inadvertently been infected, she would pass it on to future children.

Our local doctors were miraculous, caring, praying. *Some* of the specialists—not so much. If it wouldn't have been for our GP, I don't know what we would have done. He and his staff bent over backward to help.

Her symptoms started with migraines. A migraine would hit, I'd call the doctor and ask if we could come in. They never said no. Never put us off until later or another day.

"Come on in. We'll have the room ready."

She couldn't stand light or sounds, so when we arrived, they'd usher us into a patient room, lights off, shades drawn. Quiet.

Our doctor didn't know what to do some days, either. He'd try a shot that had worked for others, we'd stay until they knew it had taken effect and then he'd send us home. Usually a nurse helped us out because by that time, Jenn was very woozy and could hardly walk on her own. With me on one side and the nurse on the other, we helped her to the car.

When we got to her home, we stumbled inside.

The Lavender Co.

Interestingly, sometime during her illness, Jenn and I started a very sweet business named The Lavender Co. We made jewelry, pottery, household decor, sachets. We used lavender in everything possible!

It kept us busy and kept our minds off her illness.

We set up a booth at many indoor craft shows and outside venues. Setting up was hard work, as we had actual pieces of furniture and pillars for display and backdrops. I had purchased old screen doors to make a trifold screen backdrop that we draped with sheer fabrics.

Shopping for the fabrics and decor was therapeutic. Shopping therapy can be an addiction now, but indeed it was our therapy back then.

The business fed our weary hearts and souls and blessed other people, too. We loved setting up a show. Women would step away from our booth, just scanning everything. At first we thought maybe they were stealing ideas. (Oh my goodness! Other vendors would do that—walk around and shoot photos of product they could adapt to their business. We eventually realized it was sort of a compliment, so we quit getting annoyed.) I'd go ask if I could help them and they'd always say, "It's just so beautiful!"

Sweet.

Yeah. We did the same thing after we set up.

Beautiful.

Sigh.

Recovery

Skimming a journal about life during Jenn's recovery:

Faith.

Walking in the pool at exercise place. Both of us.

Faith.

Rest.

Faith.

Mayo Clinic in MN

12/8/2003: Notes from Mayo Journal:

Jenn and I are in the Admissions waiting area at the Gonda Building and it's about 10:30 a.m. As we walk in, I feel peace—it's a beautiful building—stunning marble everywhere.

We settled in for a long wait—people had warned us about that. Someone was playing a piano—the melody drifted around us. Comforting. From the sound, I can tell it's a grand piano. Whoever is playing is very good.

Jenn forgot her records in the car, so I walked out to get them. As I entered the elevator, a young man who was already on, greeted me with a cheery "Good Morning!" As the doors closed behind me, I turned to him and said, "You're chipper this morning!" He said, "I ought to be. My blood work is done!"

God's gonna do great things here!

12/9/2003: Day 2 - Mayo Journal:

We're in!

If you've been to Mayo, you know that you check in and wait. And wait.

You wait to find out when your appointment is. You wait to find out where it is. Many were being told to come back later—to *get* an appointment, so we were blessed to even have one.

Neither of us slept much—especially Jenn. Her symptoms were getting worse, but she could still use the whirlpool.

Not knowing what is wrong with her is like fighting an unseen foe. How can you fight if you don't know what you're fighting?

I don't want to think anymore.

Blood tests. Colonoscopy. EKG. The testing for many diseases because of her symptoms and I guess ruling out many things—ruling out lupus, ruling out autoimmune bowel disease, ruling out chronic Lyme.

The symptoms are very uncomfortable. And the tests even more so—blood in the bowels, night sweats and shivers, blood pressures, migraine tests.

This is a roller coaster that we ride up and down. With each new suggestion of what it might be, my thoughts move to what *that* disease would be like. What is she going to have to go through? How is it going to affect her quality of life? Her marriage with Josh? Our emotions flew up in joy and relief, and just as fast, plummeted in disappointment and fear.

I spent a lot of time waiting for Jenn as she went through test after test after test. Several places I especially remember. One was more like an indoor conservatory, several tall trees planted directly in pots in the floor. People occasionally walked through, but most of the time it was me and my book. Funny. I remember the book—*Big Fish* by Daniel Wallace. As I was sitting there thinking, reading, praying, a leaf fell from the tree I was sitting under. It silently released from the tree and the whole earth seemed to hold its breath. It hit branches and other leaves, clicking and scratching its way through the maze until at last it was free—floating silently once again. It landed on the carpet with a loud sigh.

Profound moments.

Jenn and I ate lunch in one of the buildings. Subway sandwiches. We walked to a piano perch—the only name I can think of for it, as seating was right next to another piano. A black man approached the piano and started playing. How did he know we needed serenading?

Things like this happened everyday. I would like to think people were positioned all over the building to sooth our stay.

Since Jenn didn't feel well she spent more time in the room but encouraged me to go out and explore.

The artwork there is unmatched—a museum of very high quality—making anyone's stay there more pleasant. I have photo after photo.

Buildings, too. Amazing architecture.

(But now, in looking over the photos, I feel nauseous.)

Back home from Mayo. I don't know if we have any more answers now than we did before.

Mayo Clinic - Again

3/10/2004:

The doctor, this time at Mayo Clinic, was a woman. She went through the blood test results with us. No parasites, no infection. CAT scan – no abscesses, no inflammation. Large bowel normal. Small bowel normal.

Results. Her word: "reassuring."

Continue on meds. Rest. Eat a balanced diet. For fatigue try Tylenol PM. Exercise.

THEY DIDN'T KNOW EITHER.

Ortho-Bionomy

My dear sister has a friend who ministers in Ortho-Bionomy. I say "ministers" because she is very intuitive and spiritual. She listens both to the Lord and to the client's body.

I describe Ortho-Bionomy as passive chiropractics, but that is just my description.

This is from their website www.ortho-bionomy.org - "The

practitioner uses gentle movements and positions of the body to facilitate the change of stress and pain patterns. A strong focus is placed on the comfort of the individual, no forceful movements are used."

It's hard to describe, but when you are being worked on, you barely feel it. The practitioner moves your body in ways that are naturally comfortable for your body. Example: does your neck naturally drift to the right or to the left?

Again from the site, " ... very effective in helping alleviate both acute and chronic pain and stress patterns ... "

Jenn and I started driving the two hours there each way once a month, if I remember correctly.

I don't remember how many trips we made but at a certain point, Jenn was moving well, and her migraines were much better.

We give Ortho-Bionomy and my sister's friend credit for helping Jenn recover. Our doctors prayed with us and loved us. We did water therapy for balance. But when I ask Jenn now what made the difference in her recovery, she said, "Don't own West Nile. Don't say, '*My* West Nile' or '*My* fibromyalgia.' Don't let it become your identity."

3
ME

Living a Lie

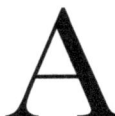gain, the journals don't lie. They tell all that I was willing to puke out on the page.

But, I was *living* a lie.

I had been bitten by the network marketing bug: "I'll make so much money!"

During all this—through Jenn's illness and Mom's recovery from a broken hip—I was trying to sell vitamins (good products—but you were forever having to add to the downline to replace the ones who got smart and quit), baskets (same as above—beautiful products, but how many baskets can you really use?).

I was always listing people's names to phone, taking notes from conference calls, adding up if I bought this many cases, it would help my bottom line. Adding in family members to my downline so it looked like I was building (I never added my pets!). And buying those family members' products so it would add up to my bigger check.

Do gamblers, when they win big, ever add up all they dropped in the slot machines or shoved across the table to the dealer? Then subtract to find the net winnings? I didn't think so.

I didn't either.

I wasn't in debt before I started those businesses.

The people were great.

The products were great.

But as I look back, I must have felt like I had to prove something. I'd like to blame it on some demon, but I think it was just my own fear of failure, fear of not having enough.

Or greed.

I never asked God. Or maybe I did, and He had spoken through my husband.

I had asked Dearly Beloved if he thought I should start. His answer? "Don't do it. It never works out. It's a scam. Don't do it."

So I did.

Journals

I spent a lot of time thinking up ideas to promote those businesses.

I should have been a copy writer back then.

Maybe I was.

"Total Body Fitness and Beauty Consulting."

Uh. Right.

"Providing a system for total well being and total well-life."

"Got body fat? Alkalize it."

I'd provide a notebook and exercise, a diet plan, recipes, nutrition info. Encouragement.

For a fee.

I guess if gym and fitness instructors could do it, so could I.

But through all of Mom's health issues, Jenn's, Jeff's, I still tried to work the business.

LIST at the back of 2003-2004 Journal:
- No Booze (except on weekends!)
- Exercise more
- Laugh more
- Read more
- No TV (except movies with Jenn)
- Don't spend money needlessly
- Save more
- No more than 2 games of solitaire daily

My Sayings and Dreams

My sayings are not as good as Harriet's (you will meet her later).

Journal entry in the midst of Jenn's illness: "Lord this doesn't feel like the **good life** right now.

I had just read Ephesians 2:10 Amplified Version, "**10** For we are His workmanship [His own master work, a work of art], created in Christ Jesus [reborn from above—spiritually transformed, renewed, ready to be used] for good works, which God prepared [for us] beforehand [taking paths which He set], so that we would walk in them [living the **good life** which He prearranged and made ready for us]."

Good life?

I heard Him say back, "It depends on how you deal with it."

Before Jenn and I went to Mayo Clinic I had another dream.

I woke in the night—couldn't sleep well—then I dozed. And dreamt.

I think I was watering my potted plants. I saw a deep hole in the dirt of one of the pots and figured some kind of bug had burrowed in there. I went to move a plant above it and a plate-size spider attached itself to my hand with skinny long claws or spikes. It hurt—I felt it.

Somehow I was able to pull it out.

THAT hurt. But as soon as I pulled it out, I was fine.

I woke up and the pain was still there. I felt God was telling me that someone had a hurt or problem buried deep or was maybe hiding it. But it would be revealed and revoked. Whoever it was would be fine and healed afterwards.

That could be all of us.

Journal quote: "Forget the cake! Go for the icing!" ~ Bonnie Lacy

Journal entry: Peace—"untroubled, tranquil, fearing nothing from God (or man), contentment, assured of salvation, undisturbed well-being, satisfied."

Humor

I am reading through every page of every journal now.

Except for Harriet's quips, and my aunt's funny sayings, there is no humor.

Everything is serious.

But in digging through every page, I found the funniest little drawing picturing the backside of a person—big boots, the rumpled pants down and butt cheeks mooning with arms bent at the elbows on either side.

I think Jeff drew it.

It made me laugh back then and it made me laugh now.

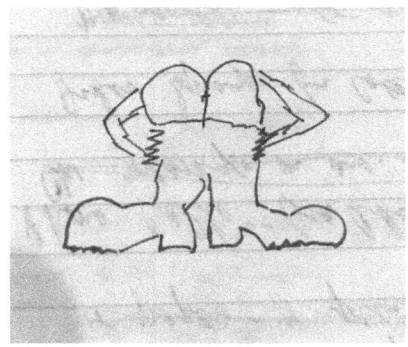

Humor heals.

THE MOVIE "GALAXY QUEST" came out in 1999, and we had a copy. I don't remember at what point in all this adventure I rediscovered it, but I do remember the day.

A day when things had crashed around me. I shoved that movie into the disk drive of my computer and played it over and over and over. I was busy, but left it playing as I stomped in and out of the office.

If it didn't make me laugh, at least it made me smile.

That's important.

Fears

Fear of failure
    Fear of looking stupid
    Fear of debt
    Fear of being found out
    Fear of no money

Getting Stuck for Months

In writing this book, I realize how stuck I was.

Every time I went to Jenn's or talked to my sister, I'd have to puke out the same story.

I'd get angry over something that had happened, or was done to me, said to me, or how I was wronged, and I would have to regurgitate it over and over. I remember doing it. I remember feeling it. It was almost like I couldn't stop. I just repeated it over and over and over again.

"He didn't say hi to me."

"I'm not wrong, they are."

"This and that and this!"

"I don't understand what I did. It was their fault."

"They didn't need to say it that way."

Awful.

And I'd go off on a tangent.

I can't imagine being the one who had to listen to this muck. It was almost like when an elderly person tells the same story over and over again. "Did I tell you about ... do you remember the time ... ?"

Over and over.

As I began to heal, I got to the point where I recognized what I was doing. Before, it had taken me months to realize I was on an endless loop. I'm not kidding. It would take me months to get off that icky merry-go-round.

It began to lessen—to maybe weeks, and then finally a couple days and now hopefully it takes me less and less time —maybe a couple of hours. Sometimes I don't even trigger. Sometimes the things that used to set me off don't even bother me.

And I am so thankful to God for that.

I find it fascinating to explore the invisible world around me. You'll know that by reading some of my fiction. I love to write about angels or demons and those realms. The more I learn about that world, the more fascinated I become.

For I know now that anger attracts demons. There is even a color they see in that realm and they gather in. All it takes is for one to tap me on my shoulder or insert a thought like, "Your husband didn't even see you," or "He doesn't care," or "He said that to make you mad."

And I'd bite.

Hard.

It was a runaway.

I'd go off full steam, spewing and crabbing. If I could have seen into that invisible world, I think I would have been terrified at what would then gather around me. With each word or phrase, a new demon would draw in and another and another until there must have been a mob of them, listening, tapping into my anger, inserting their talons into my thinking.

Icky, huh.

As I've healed, I've learned a few things.

What surrounded me affected my whole environment. My relationships. They affected everything I did. They affected everything I thought.

I dictated part of this book and as I speak this now, I am incredulous I even survived, when I think about all that was really going on in the physical and the spiritual world together.

I am so thankful to God.

And I'm thankful to Jeff for getting in my face and telling me I was angry—but I'm getting ahead of the story. I had no idea. But I am so thankful for the people who stuck by me—for Rich, that he didn't walk out on me. For my kids, my friends, my family.

None of us is perfect, I know that. It takes recognizing what we've been doing, making a choice to be different and to heal.

I have to take responsibility for my own issues. I can't change my husband. I can't change my kids—they're adults now. I can't change my friends. I can only change me, with God's help. And I am so grateful that … I am just so grateful.

Today, when I realize I'm going into that mode of anger, I've learned to stop it. I've learned ways to get out of it. Faster and faster.

I use a special prayer that is so simple and so quick.

"Forgive me. Help me."

The moment I do that, I turn into Him—Father—and I know I'm forgiven.

At that moment I can either reframe my world and my day, or choose to continue in the garbage. When there are demons around, that's what they want me to do. So they will point me in that direction. They will try to draw me back into that spewing anger.

But it's a choice.

It's a choice to be conscious and focused.

It's a choice to either turn into God with repentance or gather in the demons.

Ick.

4

JEFF AT TEEN CHALLENGE

Denver

From January through March 2004, I got the chance to go to Denver, live with son and daughter-in-law and baby, and work on a big project that his firm had been blessed with.

For a couple years we had been suspecting that our other son Jeff, was on a different path—possibly the path of drugs—but we didn't know for sure. We just suspected that, since he didn't come home for many holidays. Rarely Thanksgiving. He did come home most Christmases, but the communication between us was difficult. He didn't return our calls.

We knew something was going on, but we didn't know how to approach him or how to deal with our concerns.

It wasn't until I went to Denver to work with Jeremy, that we found a way to connect with Jeff.

As I look back, I couldn't have planned my life any better than what God planned. He had me in Denver at the same time Jeff was deciding he needed to come clean and deal with the drugs in his life.

I felt that I abandoned Jenn, and in a way I did. She was still struggling with West Nile.

Working in Denver put me next to Jeff when he began working at Jeremy's firm, too. I thought that was odd. Jeff already had a very good job for another firm and had attained the position of Senior 3D Art Director.

But it was time. Because while I was there in Denver, things began to unravel for Jeff. I think he began to realize what he was doing to himself. Also, he saw his older brother with a wife and a child, and I feel he wanted that.

He began to be more honest about what he was doing and opted to go talk to a counselor who was connected to his firm. Evidently, Jeff's was such a big design firm that the CEOs were just fine with whatever their designers did, like drugs or booze or both, just as long as their design juices flowed. Or at least that's what I figured.

But even while he was going to the firm's counselor, he fell and used again. I got the chance to sit in on one or two appointments, and Jeff confessed. He had been lying to us, to the counselor, to himself.

He finally realized he couldn't get free from drugs by himself.

Journal Entries

We decided to look in that local area for rehab places. At one location, they showed us around the facility. It was nice and of course in Colorado, with beautiful surroundings. On the tour, the lady pointed out shelves of mugs and plates that looked like they had been hand decorated by the clients. She commented that when a client was dismissed he or she would get to take home their mug or plate they had painted, as a sort of diploma.

I'm glad I didn't open my mouth and say what I was thinking.

What was I was thinking?

Oh yea.

It would cost us $9,500-$13,500 (from their website) for a *month* there and hopefully he'd recover. And he'd get a mug? Or a plate?

She was proud of the fact that the success rate was 60%. I badly wanted to ask, "Then your failure rate is 40%?" But I didn't.

And now that Jeff has read this, he remembers the success rate as 15-18%.

Success.

You do the math to figure out the failure rate.

I googled Christian drug rehab centers online. And up popped Teen Challenge.

At about the same time Jenn must've been talking to her sister-in-law and her fiancé. *He* was suggesting Jeff go to a Teen Challenge facility. Funny thing was (I guess it's funny now), but for a period of nine months it would cost us $400 and out of that $400, they bought the guys a substantial pair of boots because they would work hard. Colfax, IA was the right Teen Challenge facility, in his opinion, as it was surrounded by nature and the building was amazing.

We visited Teen Challenge in Denver. The interesting thing was that as we walked up to the location, Jeff commented that this was the biggest drug street ever. He had seen drug deals go down there.

The street was busy, an older street. But as soon as we

opened the door to that Teen Challenge building and stepped inside, Peace hugged us. The difference between outside and inside was truly amazing.

Jeff, by that time, was willing to admit he had a problem and needed help, but he was nowhere near admitting he needed Jesus Christ in his life. He did admit to feeling the peace and that there was something different in that Teen Challenge facility. It was still expensive—$1700 a month for a year.

This place only held fourteen guys. They said it was the oldest and the largest. The guy that we talked to recommended that Jeff find a Teen Challenge center out of state. He said they wouldn't say no to him at the one in Denver, but it was usually better to go farther away from where they had actually used drugs.

Jeff and I pursued what to do next. As I'm scanning my notes from back then, we were moving towards going to Teen Challenge in Colfax, Iowa.

One note, "How can we reserve a bed?"

Our Decision Made

Once his decision was made, the to-do list grew: call teen challenge, pick up dry cleaning, send power of attorney, call for license, make haircut appointment.

Jeff got hold of my notebook one day and added to the list: get all hairs cut, go rob a bank, flunk high school. At least his sense of humor seemed somewhat intact.

The next page was a list of people he owed money to.

The main item on the list: help Jeff get free of drugs. Items we hadn't even thought about: pay his bills, move his stuff, be his Power of Attorney.

Most bills had gone to collection agencies. We began calling them, one-by-one, asking for a settlement. Would they take fifty percent of what Jeff owed if we gave them the money right then? Then forgive the rest? I learned to ask.

One man on the other end of the phone line was gruff—at first. I stuck with my request for a settlement and as he and I worked out the details, he learned more of our story. He became a friend. He became kind and encouraging to a mom who was in over her head, trying to help a son.

We didn't want to leave bills behind in Denver, so we called or visited every place Jeff might have debt. Every time, we were up front in telling the truth. Each person that we talked to was touched and related their own experience with drug abuse or a loved one's hardships. Honesty and transparency always brought ministry.

My lists were now filled with settlements, credit card payoffs, letters to credit bureaus. Lining up things like Social Security cards, birth certificates, life insurance, admission sheets, school transcripts. Clean out Jeff's apartment. Load all. Move it home.

It's funny when I read the journals now. The fact that I was preparing to go back to Mayo with Jenn, noting when mom would be dismissed from the home after her hip break and checking on the Social Security office for Jeff kind of stopped me. And there's a notation Friday night to go out with friends. Dye hair. Like all of this is just normal and I guess it was for then.

I guess it was.

Jeff to Teen Challenge

The day arrived to take Jeff to Colfax. He and I drove to my sister Jan's house in Shelby, Iowa, stayed overnight, and the next morning, we took Jeff the rest of the way. I can't describe the feeling I was having as I drove, even though Jan and I were distracting each other with conversation.

I was scared for Jeff. Nervous. Would he be okay? A mom never quits worrying.

In the back seat, what was Jeff thinking? He had given up an amazing job. He was giving up his freedom for at least a year. Friendships. Even family for the time being. His belongings.

When we arrived, I can't remember who greeted us, even though through the rest of that year and a half, I came to know those people very well.

Somebody took Jeff and checked him in and I'm sure checked for drugs.

And somebody else took Jan and me around to give us a tour of the facilities. It was an amazing old building with an interesting history.

And then it was time for us to leave.

To leave Jeff.

He was safe.

And I knew where he was.

5

MOM

Assisted Living

By this time the three of us—Mom, my sister and I—had made a decision that Mom needed to live closer to one of us.

We had written down her wants, needs and requirements, and then as we searched out every place, had noted how each facility rated.

There was one near my sister in Iowa and one in my town just a half a block from my home. Mine won out because staff cleaned the apartment, cooked the meals, and did laundry. Also, Mom would have had to renew her drivers license to move to Iowa.

A main requirement on Mom's heart was that we girls would have our own life.

We wanted our own life, sure. But we wanted to hug hers, too.

We sold furniture that wouldn't fit the apartment.

We sold china she had painted. Lovely plates and dishes.

She had enjoyed china painting, but her eyes had worsened, so it was no longer something she could see to do.

We gave away a lot of her possessions. When someone bought and carried off a large wing-back chair, we made sure to have plenty of odds and ends sitting on it so they had to take the chair and whatever clutter we had gathered on the seat. Every little bit helped to clear out her home!

Measure her new closet. Measure her long clothes. (Maybe you don't know—she was short.)

Sell her house.

Insurance.

Electricity.

Water.

WHEN WE WERE SEARCHING out places, we wanted to live her life with her.

Now that she was living a half block away, she wanted to live her life and mine too. Just being honest.

JOURNAL LISTS: care plans, fifteen minute exercise, movie night, activities, locks on cupboards.

THE TOUGH DAYS when I had to confront Mom about driving, or eliminating some of her food supplements, I wanted my body to hurt just as much as my heart, so I ran around the block. Past the old ball diamond, through the park. I was a lot younger then, but I still stumbled in the dark, into holes and over twigs. By the time I stopped in front of my house, my heart still hurt, so I ran around again. And again. Exhausted, in tears. My body still didn't hurt on the outside enough, but I couldn't move anymore.

My journals turned into to-do lists: bank, call Assisted Living, call my Dearly Beloved, groceries, get meds, discontinue softener salt deliveries.

List Mom's possessions to give away. Ask people what they want.

Still at this point, lists of possible causes for Jenn's illness.

Set up Mom's banking business. Copy her address book into computer.

Will Mom want her boombox anymore?

In the middle of *my* list was Mom's scribbled handwriting—someone had given us their address and email and she wrote it down on my notebook.

My handwriting is beginning to look just like hers.

Lung Cancer

Notes from my journals—doctor appointment in a week or more, breathing machine. Do as much as we want to do. Feeding tube. Living will. Do not resuscitate.

Mom's lungs were not functioning properly—in fact the lower right lung was not functioning at all. She had a bad cough. A pulmonologist did a scope and breathing test, which were tough on her. He tried to do multiple biopsies and drain off fluid. When he had it tested, it all came back negative as far as cancer. He could never get through to get a true biopsy, though. The doctor, who had an accent like the assistant in the movie "Short Circuit," said "it is a puzzlement." And a big problem. He didn't want to do surgery so he could find out.

Due to diabetes, she was now on insulin and I learned to do the shot also.

Everyday, when I walked back and forth to Assisted Living from home, I'd see a single leaf drop in front of me, from a tree. Drifting, dancing, falling. Kept hearing the words, "letting go."

QUOTES from my journal the year after she died. 8/16/05: "Security is mostly a superstition. It does not exist in nature nor do the children of man as a whole experience it. Avoiding danger is no safer in the long run than outright exposure. Life is either a daring adventure, or nothing." ~ Helen Keller, 1880-1968, Blind/Deaf Author and Lecturer.

QUOTE FROM BETTE MIDLER: "That laughter feels really good. That there's a lot of conscious, tangible evil afoot in the world. That the planet will always go on. That you can find peace in nature. That music has great charm and is a great communicator. That dancing is good for the soul. That beauty is very healing and great for the spirit. That you gotta eat a little dirt before you die. That payback is a bitch. And that no matter who you are, there is no free lunch."

DO NOT WORRY ABOUT whether or not the sun will rise; be prepared to enjoy it. ~ Anonymous

10/12/2005: "Whatever course you decide upon, there is always someone to tell you that you are wrong. There are always difficulties arising which tempt you to believe that your critics are right. To map out a course of action and follow it to an end requires ... courage." ~ Ralph Waldo Emerson, 1803-1882, Poet and Essayist.

10/18/2005: from Clay Times Magazine—"'Refraction' can mean the ability to do work or withstand very high temperatures. Refraction also refers to the dispersing of light in myriad directions. 'Flux' in ceramic terms, is the melting agent, essential to the formation of glazes and the transformation of clay into ceramic material. 'Flux' also signifies change, sometimes dramatic and energetic change."

Walker

Journal entry December 12, 2002:
 "There is a chance the meds for pain are causing nausea."
 What?

I am digging into a certain journal and am puzzled by the above entry. It might be about Jenn, but another page or two further in gives a med schedule—1/2 pain—every two hours. We didn't do that for Jenn.

Then it hit me!

Mom broke her hip back then, and I had completely forgotten about it in the chapter lineup for this book.

So in the middle of Jenn's illness, Mom broke her hip and since my sister was still employed full-time, I went to live with Mom for three months and helped pack her house to move to Assisted Living in my town.

I remember now.

So, when the phone call came, I was at the grocery store, working.

I abandoned Jenn to go take care of Mom.

JANUARY 7, 2003:

I wrote in my journal that Mom said, "Time to get the weeds gone."

It's January. Hopefully the weeds are gone!

She was not herself from pain, confusion from meds.

One evening as we were watching the suppertime news, she shuffled to her walker, brought it to me and sat down on the little hassock right in front of me—blocking my view of the TV as I sat on the sofa! I don't think she was feeling confused that time. She was feeling better and getting ornery!

Marriage Long Distance

Memories are starting to come back to me as I dig through a journal of lists.

Do this.

Find that.

Call Assisted Living to have the cabinets lowered—remember, Mom is short!

Business list: call, email.

Call Assisted Living for Mom's new address.

Move in date: February 10, 2003.

Rich was still hauling classic cars for our business—Rich's Classic Transport. I was at Mom's home for around three months. I remember escaping back to Osceola, our home, once or twice for a weekend when my sister, Jan, could come stay with Mom.

When I couldn't get home, Rich and I met at a restaurant in Kearney. He'd be driving near and stop. We'd meet and have a meal together. He'd dump the mail out on the table and we'd sort through it and do any business that needed to be taken care of as we waited for our food.

Long distance marriage.

Letter to Mom

After Mom died, I wrote her a letter and sent it to my sister and my kids. Here it is:

∽

"Dear Mom,

I miss you so much. I don't know how to write this.

You gave me life and for that I thank you.

I am so grateful for the time we had together. For how close we were. You always listened. And heard me.

You always supported whatever I tried to do. Even when you still worked full-time. You were an awesome nurse and it was an honor to be able to work with you when I was in high school. I experienced more than just "Take Your Kid To Work Day."

There were times in high school, because of my over-commitment that I wanted to stay home from school—play hooky and sleep. But you wouldn't let me. I thought then you were mean. I cried, but I went. You were trying to teach me responsibility and to push through. I see that now. I'm still learning to push through.

You were a good mom. You loved us so much and I felt that. Until the very end.

Mom, I have regrets about the last few years. About when I had to take away your independence in your driving. It was so hard and you were so mad at me. If other people could have heard us on the phone that night, they wouldn't have thought much about it, but I felt like we were yelling because we never talked to each other like that. I got angry when you sneaked the keys and drove anyway. I can't say I blame you. Now *I* was the parent. I'm sorry I hurt you. Like your wants and needs didn't matter anymore. I just did what I felt was best. For you.

I have regrets about not being there enough. Especially when you couldn't drive anymore. I'm sure you felt trapped there even though we saw or talked to each other almost everyday.

But I felt like you wanted to live your life and mine, too.

Your illness challenged me to give you care, like administering your insulin shots. You were so patient and never made me feel bad. It felt terrible to hurt you.

Dying. It was hard work. This is going to sound weird, but you did such a good job.

I love you Mom and I thank you for giving me life and the legacy of such wonderful memories. No one has all *good* memories, but I had a great childhood, thanks to you and Dad.

They tell me I have to end this with good-bye, but ... well, Good-bye Mom."

6

HARRIET

Humor Expert

Harriet was my humor expert and moral support group all rolled into one cute little old lady of over eighty years. She walked with a cane and a limp. She had a curved back so when she took a step it was kind of a roll up to the next step.

She'd been married twice as far as I knew.

We were friends because a neighbor had suggested that maybe I could help drive Harriet to her doctor and eye appointments.

Okay.

I didn't have anything else going on, right?

We'd go to the hairstylist in the small town just south. Or pick up groceries at the store down the street. Sometimes she would go in with me but as she grew older she waited in the car while I went in with her list.

She'd send me in to buy her bottle of bourbon. Shhh.

She never had kids but saw a niece and two nephews maybe once a year.

Her one-liners kept me chuckling. I got so I would take my notebook with me to write down what she said, wherever we limped along. I called them Harriet-isms.

When I first started to drive her places, I always wanted to help her walk, take her by the arm. She was so stubborn, she'd resist.

I finally told her I wasn't going to do that anymore. "If you want help, you have to grab my arm. If you fall, it's your fault."

That way I didn't get into trouble. I was becoming more like her.

I found out early on that you didn't preach to her either. Even writing that now makes me chuckle. She put me in my place right away. But one day I went over to check on her—she'd always have me sit down across a little table from her matching wing chair, after I got my own tea. That day she told me she'd just been telling God what a good job He had been doing lately.

Whew!

She didn't even duck when she said that! She had a better relationship with Him than I thought.

She'd always talk about her growing up years and her family when we'd have tea. Her parents, her siblings. I'd hear the stories over and over and I never got tired of them. Her dad had been a druggist turned farmer and she always wondered at that—why he quit being a druggist and took up farming. She also listed her siblings—five altogether.

After chatting awhile about her life and family, she'd look straight at me and say, "Don't undersell yourself. Think well of yourself—nurture yourself." Always what I needed to hear.

She chattered all the time, I suppose she was glad to have

someone to talk to, but occasionally she'd stick in a word she knew I'd never use. Like "magnanimous." Haha. I had to look it up in the dictionary just now. Who uses words like that except a well-read former school teacher?

After our errands, we'd stop at the local cafe which she had never stepped foot in—it had always been the country club, where she and her friends played golf. She loved the cafe and saw so many people she had once known. Every Monday we had bean soup—her new favorite. "We hold court," she'd say.

New word. Simpatico. "Agreeable. Being on the same wavelength."

One day as we were doing our version of the two step—her right foot and my right foot, stepping at the same time—she said a word in a sentence.

I knew she was waiting. I said the first thing that came to mind. "That's not a word. You made that up!"

She was ready. "It is too. It means ... " She even used it in a sentence! Always the teacher.

I can't remember the word!

I wish ...

Another day at the cafe, an older gentleman sat down beside her and electricity buzzed between them.

He said something like, "Maybe I should stop by sometime." Chuckle, chuckle.

I think she replied, "I'll leave the porch light on for you."

They both knew it'd never happen.

But the delight on both faces was pure enchantment to me.

I think I grinned the rest of the week, and that was on a Monday!

If she forgot something, she'd laugh and say, "I wonder

where Harriet went." Or, "Do you have anybody as nutty as I am?"

I threw out a boxelder bug that was crawling on one of her prized paperweights. "Honey, that was part of the decorations!"

If you're bored with my memories of Harriet, you can skip this. I'm having too good a time reliving her wit!

Funny lady.

Perfect Timing

Right smack dab in between a trip to Mayo Clinic with Jenn to still find out what was wrong … and Rich's accident, Harriet and I had an outing and she was my much-needed humor. We were ready to go to her hair appointment, I think. "I've got me. I've got you and I've got my own hair."

One day the mail was very heavy. She started laughing. "I think I'll roll my window down and throw some out—one-by-one." She knew she'd get a rise out of me. Ornery lady!

She'd go through her mail in the car on our way to the hairdresser. One letter spoke of an annual drive for money—"annual drives come daily." If the envelope said something like "important information inside," Harriet said they wanted money. "Oh, is there a check made out to me? That makes it more fun!"

"I need some quiet time. How's your jail?" She meant our county jail, but I was already in my own prison of anger.

If she only knew.

She reminisced about life after her first husband passed, when she traveled a lot by herself. I asked her where she got the courage.

"I wasn't thinking—just doing."

MOM MOVED in across the street at Assisted Living. "It's going to be tough to live your own life." Harriet literally faced me in her passenger side seat. "You'll have to learn to lie."

Gasp.

"LIDGTTFTATIM." This was a plaque that she gave me. Just that. Interpretation: "Lord I do Give Thee Thanks For The Abundance That Is Mine." I had crawled under her bed to search out a hearing aid battery, and when I stood back up, I saw it hanging on her wall. She told me all about it and promptly took it off the wall and gave it to me. I learned not to comment on much. She was clearing out and would grab the item and hand it to me.

But, Lord I do Give Thee Thanks for The Abundance That Was Mine through knowing Harriet!

Magnanimous woman!

PART II
RECOVERY

7
BRIDGE TO RECOVERY

Letter to Anger

Recently, I listened to a podcast on writing, www.thecreativepenn.com, and Joanna Penn had as her guest Orna Ross, www.ornaross.com. They were talking about something Orna does at her workshops which is to have the participants write a letter to money. "Tell money what you think of it."

So I did that. I wrote a letter to money doing exactly that. It was very uncomfortable at first, writing to a piece of paper—a dollar bill—or chunk of metal—coins. But memories flooded in and I wrote those down and before long, I had a whole letter ... to Money. I capitalized it because by this time it was a person ... almost. My attitude surprised me. It's all there, in black and white. (It'll be in a book, *Cash Envelopes*, due out in 2018.)

Joanna took this practice of writing a letter to money a step further.

I am a big fan of Joanna Penn's fiction, but as an author, I also love her books on writing and the entrepreneurial life. One I am reading (along with about six other books) is The Healthy Writer written by Joanna and Euan Lawson. In it they address many health issues, but she applies what she learned from Orna Ross and wrote a letter to sugar.

I know.

It starts: "Dear Sugar, We're breaking up. You're an addiction, and you're killing me slowly, sweetly—"

So. I did it too. But I wrote a letter to Anger.

DEAR ANGER,

I am done with you. I get angry just thinking about how you have used me. Abused me.

I used to partner with you, throw parties with you. We had a great time—or should I say we carried on together famously.

I have to be honest. You used me, but at the same time, I used you. I rode the high of your emotion for days, weeks, even months over one injustice. And I found that with you, I got a lot done—vacuuming, screaming, scrubbing sinks, cussing, walking, or honestly—stomping. I wrote words in journals that people should never, ever read, but my word count exploded. All because of you. You pushed me beyond what I thought I could do, should do. We soared together.

You gave me power beyond anything I'd ever experienced. I had courage to confront and condemn because of you. There were days when I didn't care what others thought of me. I did what I wanted, when I wanted.

I stood on my own.

But. You have tried to break up any and all relationships that are dear to me.

You have tried to ruin my health and rob me of any joy I might have.

You have wasted my past and tried to block out my future.

Anger, I am through with you.

You will no longer rule my life, my emotions, my finances, my love life, my ministries, my friendships.

Just because some hard things have happened in my life, doesn't mean that I need to embrace you and invite you in.

You no longer own me.

Bonnie

Strange?

Try it.

Use whatever seems to rule your life.

Shopping?

Booze?

Pleasing others and not God?

I don't get it either. How can writing a letter to something free you?

But it does.

It's a start, a beginning.

There are still things and times to work through.

At first, the hardest thing for me was to stop. To recognize when I was angry. It had become such a part of me that I felt like it *was* me. I can't believe it now, but I would rant for months because of what one person had said or done.

I don't think I knew who I was without anger. It had become such a part of me that I didn't realize it had infested my bones, my peace, my health, the very depths of who I was.

After breaking up with Anger, I had to discover me.

Angels and Anger

If I could have only seen into the invisible world during my mess—during those years—when I spewed out those slimy words.

Father, let the Angels help me see. Aim that panoramic camera into my own face, picking up all the vile sparks flung at people, at things. Help me see.

I'm sure my face was a give-away. Eyes squinted. Mouth in a thin line. Chin jutted out. My shoulders tight and hunched. If this is a character sketch, then there it is.

Inside, every organ had to tense, anticipating the words that would be released into the atmosphere.

My mouth opened and all creation ducked because it had experienced my words before.

And the angels stepped back.

Re-reading the above line, "And the angels stepped back," makes me shudder.

There are many things going on in the invisible world that I don't yet fully understand, but I know we definitely feel the emotion of another person—whether it's anger or joy. Have you ever bumped into someone who affected you in a negative or positive way?

I experienced this in a bookstore one day. I was happily letting myself shop each section, coffee in hand, just enjoying books! I was in the Christian section, specifically the Bibles, when a woman and I met. I was passing to my left and she was moving to her right. Normally, you would smile and maybe excuse yourself, give them space or they would go around you, but she put off some kind of aura in an unkind way.

She never looked at me, but above me. By the energy she

gave off, she almost spoke the words, "Move! Get out of my way!"

That's the way it felt.

I didn't let it affect me, although I had never experienced anyone's circle of energy quite to that level before. I didn't say anything to her, but I was amused at the same time, because it seemed so absurd when all she needed to do was smile and excuse herself, move around me. I do remember chuckling at the time, which probably didn't help. I would have moved if she'd have asked!

Thinking back to times when anger controlled *me*, I *know* people next to me had to feel it. And the more tangible angels have become to me, I know they had to feel it too, hence they probably withdrew from me.

Just as angels seem affected by anger, I feel demons are attracted to it. What attracts them? Is there a color or energy a person puts off when they are angry that draws those demons in? I'm still searching this out, but maybe anger appears as red? I have only recently been learning about frequencies and wavelengths. This is funny, but my husband's snoring is one thing that spurred my studies. What is the frequency of *snoring*?

Back to words and anger. Not only were my surroundings and people close by affected, but I know my insides were affected. Ever feel really beat up after an argument or confrontation? What if those toxic words thrown back and forth had the power to change atmospheres or our health?

Have you heard about Japanese Dr. Masaru Emoto and his research? He "discovered that molecules of water are affected by our thoughts, words and feelings. Since humans and the earth are composed mostly of water, his message is one of personal health ... ." His book, *The Hidden Messages in Water,* presents his photographs of how crystals formed in frozen water reveal changes when specific, concentrated thoughts are directed toward them.

Check out his book.

From the front overleaf—"He found that water from clear springs and water that has been exposed to loving words shows brilliant, complex, and colorful snowflake patterns." The opposite is true—"polluted water, or water exposed to negative thoughts, forms incomplete, asymmetrical patterns with dull colors."

It is documented that our human body is made up of anywhere between 50% to 90% water. If I was to believe the 90% water, I'd be a puddle (some days, I feel like that!). NASA says 70%. Some websites recommend 50-60% (and we all know the internet is accurate—hence my range of percentages). Body organs' percentage of water: Brain 75%, Heart 75%, Lungs 86%, Muscle 75%, Liver 85%, Kidney 83%, Bone 22%, Blood 83%, Saliva 95%, Perspiration 95%

What if ... since the human body is more than half water ... when I spewed out my words of anger and spite ... what if I caused my own health to suffer?

Back to the frequency thing. What if my words had a harmful frequency, one that could resonate deep within my body, turning the water in each organ into harmful or deformed cells? Is that what autoimmune disease is all about? I'm not a scientist or medical doctor. I'm just searching as much as you are for answers to health dilemmas. But water is a big part of our thinking process, our digestion. Even our joints need water to stay cushioned.

Does *love* attract angels?

If my angry, putrid words push away the angels, draw in demons, and stir up a bunch of nasty responses in my body, isn't it time to find a way to *attract* angels—not demons?

Again, does love attract angels?

Lord, restore my soul.

8

JEFF IN MY FACE

Jeff - "You're Angry!"

When Jeff was with Teen Challenge, in 2004, he had some freedom, so we checked him out for the day to go shopping. We usually had to stop at Walmart to get some things he'd need, like deodorant and aftershave.

We climbed into the truck, and I don't remember exactly what I said to him, but he stopped me.

He said, "Mom. Mom! You're angry!"

And I proceeded to yell back at him, "I AM NOT ANGRY!"

The *fact* that I had yelled it, yelled back at me—that I was indeed very angry.

After that, I realized I needed help.

I knew I needed Jesus' help, but I didn't know what that meant, practically.

I only knew that the insides of me felt scrambled. They felt terrible, they felt puky. Sick. Like every organ inside of me had solidified and become hardened. Every piece of me—every brain cell, every heart cell, every blood vessel, every piece of my lungs.

Whatever we did after that, we probably finished his shopping and went to get something to eat. That was a big treat for him. Even though the Teen Challenge food was fantastic and healthy, he always enjoyed getting out to eat at a different restaurant. We even got approved to take out four or five guys to go with us. Teen Challenge gave me so much favor. The staff at Teen Challenge would recommend a new place for us to go and we enjoyed sampling the food.

We went to a coffee shop in downtown Des Moines, and that was fun. We had many good, good times, even though Jeff was still a student. We explored a little of Des Moines and definitely Colfax, IA.

But this day, the day that Jeff got in my face and told me I was angry, stopped me.

That day I knew something had to change.

I knew *I* had to change.

And I didn't know how.

I didn't know where to go, or what to do, but I knew that Jesus, somehow, was the answer to my freedom from anger.

Listening and transcribing these words from the recorder, I hear the birds twittering in the background. Even now as I write, the pain is real, but there is *hope* in the sound of the birds.

I had totally closed myself off from other people—my family, my friends. I knew I had stacked up every brick, slathered on the mortar of anger, to keep this wall up. I also knew that each brick had to be taken down, and it would be painful.

Jeff and Dad

6/1/2004: Journal entry:

"Lord, help Jeff deal with the disappointment from his dad not visiting Teen Challenge. Help Jeff see his dad through Your eyes. Heal them both."

9
CHRIST-LIFE

Teen Challenge is an Amazing Place

Teen Challenge is an amazing place.

First of all, they saved my son's life.

Secondly, they are in the business of restoring families.

But Teen Challenge also saved me from anger.

Through Teen Challenge, "John Marquez began leading individuals through a discipleship process he called *The Christ-Life Solution*. It was developed to help people deal with the effect of unfinished issues from their past so they could move forward into the life and freedom God intended for them. As participants began to experience dramatic life change, word spread. Soon the growing number of friends, relatives and acquaintances requesting to go through *The Christ-Life Solution* required that the materials be put into a written format so others could be equipped to lead these groups. In 1998, having been personally impacted by this process, Jim and Kathie Hobson began co-laboring with John Marquez." The Christ-Life Solution is now called The Ultimate Journey—see www.theultimatejourney.org—which is where I took this information from.

I looked into it—found the information.

But as I tried to figure out how it worked—scheduling and all that—I was terrified.

Terrified of who I had become.

Terrified of who I'd become if I *didn't* do something.

Terrified of what I'd do.

Terrified of what people thought of me, or of what people would think of me if I didn't get set free.

Terrified of what people would think of me if they knew I was in counseling. I was a woman who others came to for hugs and ministry.

Terrified of who I'd be.

Terrified if people found out the real me.

But nothing with Christ Life or Teen Challenge surprised them. The fact that I'm a mom, I'm a nice person. I look decent. I look normal. I've always been a "good girl." With all the people they'd dealt with—the people they'd set free—nothing surprised them.

They had turbo weekends, where you'd cover what the guys at Teen Challenge had done. What they had achieved over a period of weeks, maybe months, you would do in a weekend.

I'd go to Colfax, IA and stay at Teen Challenge, then attend the meetings and we'd fill out questionnaires, gather in a small group of four people.

I always found that my childhood was just sweet—not perfect, but sweet. Other people's stories, believe me, would shoot you off your chair. They didn't realize their childhood was abusive.

And again, those stories would stay within that room.

I found out that my childhood was wonderful.

I had a tree house that my uncle had built for me. I spent a lot of time in that tree house listening to the cottonwood leaves clap their hands, writing down my thoughts, listening to the birds and just *being*—staring.

At one point I had been talking with some of the students in Teen Challenge. The leaders let me talk to them, minister, nurture as I felt led. It might have been at an evening they had set up with the guys to share and we had chapel and worship — oh my goodness, to worship with those guys—wow.

The guys started talking about their childhood, their lives. Many had been *given* drugs as kids by their parents. Most had been abused by someone.

I always apologized. I wasn't abused, I didn't do drugs—ever. Maybe booze but not other drugs.

I almost made excuses for my wonderful childhood. Not almost. I did. I made excuses.

At the end of the evening, when I entered my room, I could feel Father withdraw from me.

What?

What did I say?

I had hurt my Father in Heaven's feelings by being ashamed of the good, fantastic, wonderful, beautiful childhood He had given me—that He had blessed me with—that He had chosen for me to be born into.

I cried out to him. I apologized to him.

I cried.

Even now as I transcribe this, I hear the emotion in my voice on the recording.

"I'm sorry Father. I'm so sorry."

I had a wonderful childhood and I thank God for it.

So Christ Life was the beginning of recovery from the evil anger I had let seep in.

10

TAKE CARE OF ME

Words Spoken Over Me

At some point I had been at a church and a minister spoke over me. He was always very creative and accurate.

This time he "saw" a huge steam shovel. In his vision, as I ran that piece of equipment, I was digging in too deep, taking too big of a bite out of the dirt. He said I needed to back up and readjust how much I bit off.

Journal entry: "Lord help me understand what can be fixed in the steam shovel picture and what can't, and to accept it. Give me a revelation of what I need to adjust. Please continue to work through the insurance things and help me persevere through and to keep at it. Never give up. Give me wisdom to follow through and how."

Don't know the date, but this quote is mine – "There're two

ways to look at life – go slow enough to see every ladybug on the road. Or go fast enough to see every road!"

After Effects

So much that I can't even write about. Mom. What she went through. What Jan and I went through and continued to go through.

And you know what? It doesn't matter. What matters is that we didn't quit. Mom didn't quit. She plunged through. She worked hard. She overcame death and blazed right into the Throne Room, and spent Christmas with the King. That's what matters.

I had been having trouble with my neck glands during all this. I'm not sure when they started hurting but it felt like there was a strong rubber band around my neck from the bottom of one ear down around the front of my neck and up to the bottom of my other ear. Tight. It felt like I was choking. It literally hurt like someone had their hand at my throat, choking me.

Jesus gave me a sense with all that year had presented—Jeff's addictions, Jenn's illness, Mom's illness and death—I held it all in. Not even trying to be strong, although that is a part of it. It was about not looking stupid, about not getting all slobbery, with my make-up running down my face. Or snot running out of my nose. It was about not falling apart in front of someone. And that band around my neck was the result of years of holding that jaw straight, of holding in the tears. Keeping that mouth set. Not letting Jesus help me heal. And maybe I'm that way with friends and family, too. Always the strong one. Never let down. Never let them help ME.

A FRIEND WAS ALWAYS OFFERING for me to get a soda with her. And I never called her.

Lord, help me call her. Just writing that now, brought tears. I love her and our time together, but what will "they" think if I have to ask for help?

People need to be needed. People need to know that they are helping someone. Even in having a coke together.

I HAD SO many thoughts about Mom. About our time together before she died. Of those almost two years together in Osceola. Of how I didn't spend enough time with her. Or how I didn't see her every day. How I didn't take her enough places after I took her driving privileges away.

Of how I wanted to live MY life and *she* wanted to live my life too—like I said before, but it bears repeating.

There. I said it. It's out. And it makes me cry.

Because, yes, I have regrets. We all do.

I regret that I didn't get to take her to see the Christmas lights one last time (She was too sick. She died December 5th.)

I regret I didn't take her to Jenn's to see the kitties more. She loved going there. But I knew how hard it was on Jenn. Or was it hard on me?

I regret I didn't let her rub my back more when she offered. She needed to "mother me." I didn't need it. I'm too strong. I don't need anyone's help.

Maybe you say that I shouldn't have any regrets, but I need to get this out.

All of it.

Out.

I need to have those bands around my neck released. Gone.

And right now I am a mess. Ick. Snot running … well I'm sorry, but you get the picture.

I think that those "regrets" are really a sadness. I'm sad her life is over. I'm sad that I won't ever get another chance with her.

I am going to be BRUTAL, but in the scheme of things, would I have played it any different if I had had another chance? Would I have learned my "lesson"?

11

COUNSELING

Becoming Me

I connected with a counselor in Stromsburg—a town close by.

She definitely helped with the grief over losing Mom—I was struggling in doing all the things my sister and I had to do and releasing all the things we had to release.

But I think that next to the anger (though I don't think there was much anger about Mom), I was missing her. Grieving her loss. I don't think anger had any roots there, that I know of right now.

The counselor recommended books.

She let me talk.

She asked me questions.

And it definitely helped talking through the grief.

Things my sister and I had to do: taking Mom's car keys from her, packing up suitcases and suitcases of Mom's food supplements—bottles and bottles, moving her from her beautiful home in Holdrege, NE to assisted living in Osceola, NE.

All of that.

Watching her die.

Watching her physically die.

The counselor talked me through all of that.

My sister and I had spent the morning with her in her apartment, holding her, loving her. Watching over her. Jan was supposed to leave for home, but an ice storm kept her there.

As soon as we took a break for lunch and brought our plates into the room and were just sitting down to eat, we kinda glanced over at Mom and my sister said, "Mom just took her last breath."

There she was.

In heaven.

Her body was still there but Mom had gone to heaven.

The counselor talked me through all of that.

Talked me through anger about things that had gone on with the farmhouse we still owned.

She was definitely a part of many people who prayed for me, prayed over me, who helped me puke out my ugly soul.

She helped me take bricks down. Helped me scrape them off—that yucky mortar—and clean them up. We made beautiful pathways and patterns with all the cleaned up bricks.

A wonderful tribute to Mom's life. I'm not sure where those brick paths are, or where they're leading, but I'm doing my best to seek them out.

I'm trying to figure out who I am without the anger. I am trying to build *my* desires back into my life.

It's like a river channel—as floods come, or drought—the river follows new channels. It's difficult to get back to the original channel. Maybe the river never needs to get back to the original, but instead finds the *right* channel with the rocks, trees, and river bed that are currently in its path.

Our life is like that, except we can change things back—if we want. But as the situations change in our lives (like needing to be caregiver), those things change us and help shape who we are and are to become. So sometimes we never want to get back to the original because we have become someone else.

With me, it seems selfish to embrace my desires, but it's because I am becoming the real me again. And it feels good.

Yes, there are struggles—just as the river goes through change. It has to carve out new channels—sometimes through stone. But it can be done. The struggles are mostly within ourselves—new paradigms about who we *really* are. Who God really made us to be.

The *real* original channel.

There are struggles with our families because of the shifts, but once they know what we want, they want it for us, too.

So maybe I'm not selfish. It just feels that way as I take back as much of the original river that I need back in my life. I'm shifting channels, and that sometimes causes others to have to shift also. They don't like that!

But I'm carving out my new river bed edged with beautiful brick pathways.

12

STRONG TOWER

Prayer Tunnel

I had been through counseling and Christ life, but now it was time to get down and dirty.

Jeff was still in Teen Challenge, so I met my sister and her friend at the church in Omaha where he had been attending and they had a prayer tunnel set up for the end of the service.

Prayer tunnel, ha.

That means that all the people on the prayer team line up on both sides of the aisle, and whoever wants prayer walks in between them. So as you're walking down the aisle, there are people on both sides of you that can reach out and touch your shoulder, your arm, your head and pray for you.

But that day, I wasn't sure I wanted to do that. Oh, I wanted to get free of all the junk.

But.

The emotion in me from the grief, the anger, the fear—everything had bottlenecked at my throat. And I knew that if somebody touched me in just the right way or said just the right words, I would burst into tears. And then I would be a soppy, snotty-faced, mascara-smeared person in about two seconds.

Part of me wanted to run away. I knew some coffee shops close by so I could hide. What would *you* want to do when you're faced with emotional chaos? Definitely not walk through a prayer line and get all messy faced.

We met my son there—Jeff and some guys from Teen Challenge. I wasn't going to get all messy faced in front of them. I don't even want to do that in front of my sister.

But as I stepped into that prayer line, I felt emotion rising. I can feel it now. I don't remember every word spoken over me or prayed over me, except for one man.

By the time I reached him, I was bent over, sobbing. And he must have taken one look at me and groaned in the spirit.

Groaning and groaning.

He reached out to me and touched my shoulder. The only words he said that I remember are, "He is your Strong Tower." Those are the only words I have from him.

I probably could've collapsed right there in that prayer line, but there were people behind me. They weren't pushing me forward, but they needed to keep the prayer line moving, instead of having to step over a sobbing woman. They weren't gonna let the soppy face lady stop the whole thing. They probably should've picked me up and moved me. There should have been a sign, "In case of sobbing woman, move her to the side of the prayer tunnel." That would've been a good idea.

Because I remember I just wanted to lie down by that guy's feet—because he got it. He got the pain, he got the tears, he got the emotion. And he didn't even know who I was. He hadn't even asked me a question. He just knew.

I made it to the end of that prayer line.

I remember seeing a young woman hit the end and crawl over to the wall and just huddle there in a fetal position and sob.

I wanted to do that so badly.

But people were with me and they were watching me. I felt I had to buck up and put on a show.

I had to impress.

I had to look good.

I had to be that stalwart person.

Because everybody always came to *me* for help.

I was always too strong to ask other people for help.

Not anymore.

13

JOY - OR LACK OF IT

Busted at the Bank

You know how you remember a moment in time that is clearly cemented in your memory?

Like the birth of a child.

Or a time when someone said something nice or did something nice, you remember it forever.

This day wasn't a nice memory.

But this day was the beginning of my turnaround into new life, into freedom.

I had gone to our bank in Osceola to do some business, but what I remember very clearly, is that I was fuming inside and I don't think it was anything that anyone had said or done on that day. It was all of those things on top of each other: the accident, the illness, mom, Jeff.

I hear the emotion in my voice on the recording, as I transcribe right now.

I was so angry.

As I went into that bank and tried to smile at people, I must have looked awful.

My smile must have looked like a grimace.

Or my smile must have looked like a face in a horror movie. Grrr!

A scowl.

The face of a person that was either going to cry ... or kill.

That's how I felt.

As I greeted people, that scowl, that anger must have come out through my eyes.

The teeth I smiled with were probably bared, as I hissed, my ears flat. All of those signs you think of when an animal is ready to strike.

I remember thinking as I put my paperwork down on the counter in front of the teller, "Who would want the Jesus that they see on my face today?"

Yeah.

Because my "Jesus" that day was full of hate, full of anger, had already progressed from offenses, bitterness, resentment, anger, rage, to murder.

If anybody had gotten in my face that day, called me out on something or addressed me in a strange way—called me a name, looked at me sideways, I would have murdered.

With my tongue or with my hand.

Was it that bad?

Yeah.

And that realization, that fear, the power of that image opened my eyes.

Stopped me.

Terrified me.

I didn't know what I was gonna do. I didn't know how to do it. I didn't know who to talk to.

But once I left the bank, I went home and got out my Bible.

I opened it up to the Concordance and looked up every single verse on joy I could find, that I could understand. I tapped those verses out on my computer—a page-full or more. I printed off ten copies—I don't know why—I'm only one.

I took them with me everywhere I went. Everywhere.

I had an appointment at the doctors office sometime after that, and I had them with me—I don't know why. I guess I needed them to look at constantly. I took them in. We started talking and I think I must have told her what had happened in the bank. And she said, "Oh my gosh, I need those verses."

I gave her one.

"Can I make a copy of this?"

"Yeah. It's the Bible. It's Scripture."

She left me in the exam room, ran out and made copies for everyone in the office.

Scriptures on Joy.

As I recorded this—walking—you can hear my emotions rise. You can hear my footsteps on the pavement.

I don't know what I did with the other copies—probably gave them to my kids, maybe found some other poor blokes or victims to give them to. Brought them home—hugged them.

But I know that first of all, in the act of digging them out of the Word, then tapping them out on the computer, and saying them—speaking them out, they did something in me.

I know they did a healing in me that day.

I don't know how it works—it's one of those mysteries. Speaking them out, how the truth can set somebody free.

HERE IS the list of verses, exactly as I typed in 2005.

FEB. 14, 2005 – Joy (I know, it should be on love!)

NEHEMIAH 8:10 – "Then (Ezra) told them, Go your way, eat the fat, drink the sweet drink, and send portions to him for whom nothing is prepared; for this day is holy to our Lord. And be not grieved and depressed, for the joy of the Lord is your strength and stronghold."

PSALM 16:11 – "You will show me the path of life; in Your presence is fullness of joy, at Your right hand there are pleasures forevermore."

PSALM 27:6 – "And now shall my head be lifted up above my enemies round about me; in His tent I will offer sacrifices and shouting of joy; I will sing, yes, I will sing praises to the Lord."

PSALM 30:5 – "For His anger is but for a moment, but His favor is for a lifetime or in His favor is life. Weeping may endure for a night, but joy comes in the morning."

PSALM 51:12 – "Restore to me the joy of Your salvation and uphold me with a willing spirit."

AN OFF-SHOOT! II Chron. 20:17a – "You shall not need to fight in this battle; take your positions, stand still, and see the deliverance of the Lord (Who is) with you, O Judah and Jerusalem. Fear not nor be dismayed. Tomorrow go out against them, for the Lord is with you." Read around this.

NEH. Chapters 2 and 4 – all! Esp. 2:17-20

ISAIAH 35:10 – "And the ransomed of the Lord shall return and come to Zion with singing, and everlasting <u>joy</u> shall be upon their heads; they shall obtain <u>joy</u> and gladness, and sorrow and sighing shall flee away."

ISAIAH 51:3 – "For the Lord will comfort Zion; He will comfort all her waste places. And He will make her wilderness like Eden, and her desert like the garden of the Lord. <u>Joy</u> and gladness will be found in her, thanksgiving and the voice of song or instrument of praise."

ISAIAH 61:3 – "To grant (consolation and <u>joy</u>) to those who mourn in Zion—to give them an ornament (a garland or diadem) of beauty instead of ashes, the oil of <u>joy</u> instead of

mourning, the garment (expressive) of praise instead of a heavy, burdened, and failing spirit—that they may be called oaks of righteousness (lofty, strong, and magnificent, distinguished for uprightness, justice, and right standing with God), that planting of the Lord, that He may be glorified. And they shall rebuild the ancient ruins; they shall raise up the former desolations and renew the ruined cities, the devastations of many generations."

Matt. 13:20 – "As for what was shown on thin (rocky) soil, this is he who hears the Word and at once welcomes and accepts it with joy;"

An encouragement! Matt. 25:21 – "His master said to him, Well done, you upright (honorable, admirable) and faithful servant! You have been faithful and trustworthy over a little; I will put you in charge of much. Enter into and share the joy (the delight, the blessedness) which your master enjoys."

John 14 – all! But esp. v. 11 – "I have told you these things, that My joy and delight may be in you, and that your joy and gladness may be of full measure and complete and overflowing."

Gal. 5:22

1 Thess.1:6

Heb. 13:17

And you know James1:2-4 – "Consider it wholly <u>joy</u>ful, my brethren, whenever you are enveloped in or encounter trials of any sort or fall into various temptations. Be assured and understand that the trial and proving of your faith bring out endurance and steadfastness and patience. But let endurance and steadfastness and patience have full play and do a thorough work, so that you may be (people) perfectly and fully developed (with no defects), lacking in nothing."

That's all I had time for! Later ...

There are more—187 verses with the word "joy" in them in the King James Version, (Most of these are from the Amplified Version.) so if you need more, there are more! Digging them out is therapy—try it!

Journal Entry - Reality

5/28/2004: Journal entry:

"Carry us in Your balloon basket—up and up—in joyful abandonment. Enjoy the motion, turbulence, storms, world, sun where we go at Your whim!"

∼

6/1/2004: Journal entry:

"Lord, I sense in me that I have taken on so much that I have lost my joy—"Restore in me the joy of Thy salvation." Help me to have a happy heart and not look like I'm ready to kill someone. Help me get back into that balloon basket and see things through your eyes—a newness, a freshness, an openness. Refresh me, restore me, rebuild me! Uplift me!

∼

7/27/05: Journal entry:

What is my **reality**? That I'm alone most of the time. That I have to do most everything because Rich is on the road—home, work, food, shopping, sleep, etc.—alone.

Reality: I've had a very tough last few years.

Reality: I seem to think that I need to take care of everyone else.

Reality: Since I'm alone, I have to hire things done.

Reality: I want people to take care of me, but I won't ask.

Reality: I think I'm giving, but I'm selfish.

Reality: In being caregiver and helper, I am being self-righteous. "Oh poor me."

Reality: I am stubborn. "No, I want to be angry ten more days to make *you* feel worse." When it only eats *me* up.

7/28/05: Journal entry:

I "saw" a yoke lifted up and over my head. Heard words, "Take My yoke." Just when I was beginning to wonder, "How am I going to carry *this*?" I saw Jesus come up beside me and lift the other end over His head and shoulders. He smiled and took my hand. "Together. Equally yoked. Sharing the load." Matt. 11:29-30

14

WRITING

Writing to Healing

2/9/2005: Journal entry:
"I wonder what it would be like to write all day."
My thoughts of a wanna-be writer who struggled to find her way.

I WAS sick enough for Jenn to take *me* to the doctor. I must have had the crud (my diagnosis for everything!) and the doctor had prescribed a mega antibiotic. I had decided to let myself flake or rest, but again, was wondering what it would be like to write all day. What would it feel like to actually *be* a writer? Which is exactly what I do now, most days.

In previous chapters, I have talked about how much I've written, how many journals I have filled, but I haven't really talked about how writing has healed me.

Anne Lamott writes in *Bird by Bird,* on page 136, about

"when you give yourself permission to start writing." That's a big statement. Permission to start writing. But I notice as I dig through those journals, that I scribbled a note, "Write about keeping things bottled up or I'll explode!"

Write?

11/9/2007: Journal entry:

Our bodies reflect the pain inside, whether we are overweight or somehow diseases have overcome us. They all reflect the emotion and spirit inside. Hence my neck pain—I had been choking myself out.

JUST THE ACTION of puking it out on the page, letting my pen command and cover the whole white blank space with my thoughts is so healing. Back when I started journaling, I would scribble about something that had happened. I journaled about my life, my dreams, my plans. And actually when I first started, I wrote my prayers. Maybe I'd be praying for one of our kids and I would write on the page as the prayers poured from my heart. Sometimes I would go back and write the response or the result of my prayer for this person. But I gradually started writing more and more not only thoughts and prayers, but my dreams that I would have during the night or visions during the day. And as I wrote those down, I usually got an interpretation. So God spoke to me through the writing.

I'm having a hard time putting into words how this works for me. First I have a thought that I write down, so I have words. But at the same time I am engaged with the Father, in

Jesus, through the Holy Spirit—so I'm also writing through the Lord. I know He guides my thoughts. I know the angels bring me messages from Him.

There's something else there, in between having a thought, writing it down, and making words appear on the page as I write. I know lately as I've journaled, I'll have a question for the Lord, and I write that down. And immediately there will be a visual, a blink, a picture in my mind. And most times that will be my answer.

So to come back to the theme of this book, *Rage Rising*, every time I sit to write in a journal, when I connect with Father in heaven, he speaks to my heart—through the page and I write his answers down. With each letter, each word, each page, healing happens. I don't understand it—it's one of those mysteries. But as I rest in Him, as I engage with the Father through Jesus and the Holy Spirit, the miraculous happens on the page and His words come out. As I put my pen to the page and write, His words come out of the pen and happen on the page.

Also with the writing, when I'm confronted with a tough thing to write—whether it's tough from my own life experiences, things that happened to me, things I've done, or just what goes on in the world—as I write those things in fiction or nonfiction, I'm confronted with them. And as I confront those issues, I examine them with my pen on the page, and I find truth. If I don't get an answer right away, I pursue Him. I keep on asking and asking. I think on it daily and the answer comes.

As I am transparent, as I puke out the nastiness and publish it in a book, other people hopefully get healing too. That's why this is important—to write the words, to be open, honest. I'm reminded right now of the verse, "Faith is the substance of things hoped for, the evidence of things not seen." Hebrews 11:1.

I have faith right now that the words as they appear on these pages, through the writing of my pen, through the thoughts in my heart, through the thoughts of my Lord, *become* substance and *become* faith and *become* real and tangible. These are the things hoped for as I write—healing, power to change, peace for the reader *and* the writer.

Ending

And now, 2018. This is no journal entry.

Rich has recovered well. When it comes right down to where (Against all writing tips, I have to use this cliché.) the rubber meets the road, he is a changed man. He might put on a tough front but when we drive by *that* place along the road, he gets quiet.

We never had any interaction with the man's family, who caused the accident. I have prayed for them, but that's all.

Insurance treated it like a dinged up bumper. That's all they paid. And not to be greedy, but the accident caused heartache, trauma, loss of equipment, loss of income. I wanted to grab the adjuster by the throat and ask what they would have paid out if Dearly Beloved had died.

But thanks to God, he didn't and I have to let that one go.

MOM IS HEALED IN HEAVEN. She passed away early December and Harriet went home in January. Two of the strongest ladies (next to my daughter, Jenn, and sister, Jan) that I've gotten to know on this Earth. Since Mom was an I-want-it-done-yesterday kind of woman and Harriet was an I'm-in-charge kind of woman, I can only imagine what those two are cooking up. I'm thankful they're on God's side.

JEFF HAS BEEN many places and done many things since Teen Challenge—Hawaii and Australia as part of Youth with a Mission, become a storyteller with movie scripts *and* with wood from old buildings that have stories all their own. There are still struggles but like all the rest of us, each layer peeled back opens new wounds, but new blessings and healings.

AND JENN. I found a couple more journal entries—one from January, 2006. She'd been sick for over four years.

Jenn: "I feel like a caged-up lion and I can't get out and the cage is my body."

Me: "What is the lion doing?"

Jenn: "He's pacing."

Another entry: "If I had cancer would someone give me a spaghetti feed? When is it our turn to have good things happen? Others get new houses, jobs, babies. When is it our turn?"

A prayer I'd written: "If she is to be here with a long life, please let it happen—please let her have babies. It comes down to ... everything under heaven is Yours, Lord. She is Yours—her illness, health, babies, pain, joy ... everything on Earth is Yours. I can't see to write—" I can't read my writing at this point.

She did get a diagnosis—West Nile. After two years ...

There have been ups and downs, also, with Jenn. She and her blessed husband have five children on this Earth now. And one in heaven.

She has endured Hemiplegic migraines but has gotten them under control. She takes care of her family, bees, chickens, and Siberian Husky dogs. And years when she isn't expecting a baby, a garden with canning and juicing. God be praised.

AND ME.

There are days.

I started doodling. I let myself play. Even posted to Instagram (check out @bonlacy), which was rather gutsy of introvert me.

I took a year off from any church (I know. My pastor uncles in heaven have to be shaking their heads.)

How many of you would like to do just that—escape?

Be honest.

During that year, every Sunday I would play the piano in worship—not songs you would know, but songs from the heart of God. He showed me pictures of where to put my fingers on the keyboard and it flowed from there.

I stayed in my jammies (Another reason you'd like to stay home from church—I get it.), drinking coffee and studying all morning—my nose in the Word and in my notes. Then I'd sit back, satisfied. Finally full.

Many times while worshiping, God would tap me on the forehead, drop a memory into my imagination and challenge me to go there, knowing I needed to face it. A memory. A hurt. An unforgiven place in my heart.

After about a year, God had something up His sleeve. Spanish church.

Spanish Church

I met a Spanish speaking lady at a store I used to work at. She knew a little English and was a believer in Jesus. She taught me church words in Spanish: iglesia, alabanza. For those who are minimal Spanish speakers like me, iglesia means church and alabanza means praise. We had a great time chuckling at each other's pronunciations.

She asked if she could give me a business card for her church.

"Sure." I glanced at it and she pointed out words, the address.

We hugged as she left and I tucked it into my pocket. What would I ever need it for? But I didn't throw it away. I emptied my pockets that night and stuck the card into a little basket I keep business cards in.

I have no idea why I kept it.

But around the end of a year of having church by myself, at home—in my cave I called it—God showed me why I kept that card.

I was in the middle of worship one Sunday, when God, clear as if He was sitting in the room with me drinking coffee, said, "Go get that card."

Now I knew which one. "What card?"

He had given me a picture of it when he spoke.

"Go get the card the Spanish lady gave you about her church."

So I got it. But as I sat down on my favorite spot, I knew He was up to something. I still played dumb. "Okay. Here it is." I read it and dropped it onto the side-table.

To this day, I still have it. Really.

That was maybe eight years ago.

I still have it.

"Let's go there today."

"Wha-what?" But I knew. I knew I needed to get off that sofa, get dressed, and drive there. The card had the address, so I couldn't use that as an excuse.

You know when terror settles in and your stomach does flip-flops?

That's right. That's how I felt.

"But Lord." I put on my sweet voice. "I don't know anyone there."

That was my *first* protest?

I don't speak Spanish! Unless you count hola and taco.

Still in my sweet (read: manipulative) voice, "But I don't speak Spanish!" That would get Him.

When God has a plan, we are free to ignore it.

But.

When He has a plan, we will miss His blessings if we do ignore it.

So I went. Sounds so easy, now.

It's a thirty minute drive to the church, and I yelled all the way. Same two excuses. "I don't know anyone!" and "I don't speak Spanish."

Angels by that time were either grimacing or grinning —or both.

My stomach felt awful—like when I was in high school at my piano recital and I blanked out my song. Nothing. My stomach was tied in knots then too, until I got home and cried on my pillow.

Found the church.

Terrified.

Opened the door.

Pastor Miguel Godoy was standing just inside with a quizzical expression on his face. "Can I help you?"

English?

Stutter. Stutter. "Well, I have this card." I held up the business card. I tried to explain how I'd come to have it. I'm not sure if it made any sense.

"Well, this church moved to another address." He tapped the card. "Do you want me to tell you how to get there?"

"They moved? But what is here now?"

He glanced behind him. "We are. Centro Misionero ... " The rest was lost on me. Lots of Spanish words. "But I can direct you to where that other church is now."

What?

Lord, You didn't tell me about the address change.

The stomach butterflies had turned into writhing monsters and were doing their best to make what little breakfast I had eaten into undigested missiles that might soon become projectile.

Lord, help. What do I do?

"I uh ... I think I'm supposed to be here."

Good answer. Because as I look back, I am grieved by thinking I might never have gotten to know Pastor Miguel, his family, and others.

He helped me find a place to sit and I don't honestly remember much about that service, except at the end when a woman gave me a healing hug. She just held me. I remember the hug. I haven't seen her since.

I attended in a hit-and-miss fashion for about a month or two.

Right.

Terrified.

But, then attended every Sunday. Sometimes even Saturday night.

Amazing times that might have to be a whole other book.

God broke through my attitudes and fears. I wept every worship time, still terrified, hugging the wall. Sunday after Sunday the worship songs were the same ones, as they were just getting started in their music ministry, but God used those same songs to bypass my brain and go straight to my heart.

Breaking me.

Healing me.

Breaking me again and again.

The preaching back then. Pastor preached bilingually. Spanish. English. Spanish. English. Powerful. One Sunday, I realized that he was doing that just for me. Everyone else there was Spanish-speaking. Humbling. What a revelation. God pressed in to remind me that Jesus would have died just for me.

Now Pastor's wife, Elsa, interprets for me, which is rich with new Spanish words and meaning. It's been a joy to get to know her and Pastor so well.

God used my Spanish-speaking brothers and sisters to love me out of my attitudes, into loving myself and breaking down those bricks that I had so skillfully stacked up.

There are times still, when something—not even close to anger—rises up.

But that dark tunnel has an end and I can see a new pathway and new hope.

EPILOGUE

Tough to end a book like this, because life goes on and anger is always sneaking around the corner. As I have shared ways God brought me through, I hope you have been blessed, but even more so, encouraged in your own life.

I have permission to share these excerpts from Brené Brown's book, *Daring Greatly*, but I really hope you will pick her book up and dig in (I don't get a $20 bill for endorsing it!). In the introduction, she defines wholehearted living on page 10: "Wholehearted living is about engaging in our lives from a place of worthiness. It means cultivating the courage, compassion, and connection to wake up in the morning and think, *No matter what gets done and how much is left undone, I am enough.* It's going to bed at night thinking, *Yes, I am imperfect and vulnerable and sometimes afraid, but that doesn't change the truth that I am also brave and worthy of love and belonging.*

In Chapter 1, Scarcity, page 29, "As I explained in the Introduction, there are many tenets of Wholeheartedness, but at its very core is vulnerability and worthiness: facing uncertainty, exposure, and emotional risks, and knowing that I am enough."

It's the kind of book that I underline, doodle for emphasis, fold page corners down (illegal in some reading circles!), and soak in. I won't ever finish it, because I go back and forth—in and out—but it's one of those books you keep forever.

Writing a book like *Rage Rising* is like appearing in every place naked: in the grocery store, at church, walking down every street in every town. Admitting to some of the emotions and thoughts—in front of ... the world.

Yes, it's hard for others to know my junk, but even harder for the author—me—to go back to the journals, reviewing photos, digging into past memories.

But healing, just the same.

I realize I'm just one small person in a huge cosmic universe. What difference can writing a little book like this make?

I'm almost teary as I write this. But I do hope this book makes a difference in someone's life.

I know *writing* it has made a huge difference in mine.

Transparency.

Vulnerability.

Letting you see the real me.

And knowing.

Knowing some will criticize or laugh.

But some of you will sigh.

And hug.

And love.

In spite of.

ACKNOWLEDGEMENTS

My thanks go to so many for not only a book like this, but for saving my life. People who helped me, loved me: in spite of the revenge on my face, in spite of the words from my mouth or the look in my eye.

With each event, there were special people who took time to make sure we knew they saw us and what we were going through. They took time to give the extra kindness and words, the hugs and love.

Thank you to my Dearly Beloved, kids, grandkids and family, who didn't give up on me. My friends who still listened, even though they had heard my complaints over and over.

Thanks to my God, in Him do I trust.

Thanks always to my editor, Kathy Tyers Gillin. You see what I don't. You encourage me. You don't let me get lazy. I am a better writer because of you.

Thanks to my cover designer, Jane Dixon-Smith. I give you a title and a synopsis. You design a cover that speaks. You get it.

My beta readers. That's a whole amazing level of service, of faith. Thank you.

And my church, my pastors. You have no idea how much you give me. Next to the Lord, you are my sanctuary.

And thanks to you, Reader. There are many moments when a writer questions her work—whether to keep on writing. "What's this even for? Who really cares if I write? I should just watch TV."

But just at the right minute You, Reader, show up and encourage me, complement me. To you, your words might not be a big deal. But to me, what you say to me makes me blink, possibly tear up. But most importantly, your words make me sit back down in my chair ... and write.

Never give up. Never give in.

STAY CONNECTED

You are always welcome to email me - bonnie@bonnielacy.com with any news, questions, comments, suggestions, jokes.

Look for other titles, short stories, kids' books in the future.

Book One in The Great Escapee Series, *Released*, can be purchased here. Book Two, *Rescued*, here. Book Three will be out the end of 2018.

Cash Envelopes: You've Never Had So Much Money comes out in 2018.

Connect with me online: www.bonnielacy.com
Find my doodles and more on Instagram: @bonlacy
Twitter: @BonnieLLacy

You can sign up to be notified of new releases, giveaways, and any news I think you might be interested in - plus, get a free short story! Look for the pop-up at: www.bonnielacy.com

I greatly appreciate you taking time to read my work. If you ever want to help: 1) Please consider leaving a review wherever you bought my books. 2) Or tell your friends about it! 3) Check the shelves of your local library. 4) Use hashtags #bonnielacy whenever you talk about my books online.

Copyright © 2018 by Bonnie Lacy
All rights reserved.
Reproduction in whole or part of this publication in any form—past, present or future technology— without express written consent is strictly prohibited, except in the case of brief quotations in critical articles or reviews.
The author greatly appreciates you taking time to read her work. Please consider leaving a review wherever you bought her books. Or tell your friends about it! Check the shelves of your local library.
http://www.bonnielacy.com
Unless otherwise noted, Scripture quotes are from AMPLIFIED BIBLE, Copyright © 1954,1958,1962,1964,1965,1987, by The Lockman Foundation. All rights reserved. Used by permission. (www.Lockman.org)
Cover by JD Smith Design
Published by Frosting on the Cake Productions

Any questions about the book, or to contact Bonnie, please email:
bonnie@bonnielacy.com

ISBN-13: 978-1-943647-07-1 (Paper)
ISBN-13: 978-1-943647-08-8 (E-book)

www.ingramcontent.com/pod-product-compliance
Lightning Source LLC
Chambersburg PA
CBHW031157020426
42333CB00013B/710